Table of Cont

18-0503

Top 10 Lessons for Living a Great Life!

Here are some important life lessons kids and adults have learned. As you read each one, take a moment to think about and answer the question.

1. Believe that you are a valuable person.
How does accepting and liking yourself affect your self-esteem?

2. Show your feelings in healthy ways.
How does this affect your relationships with friends, family and others?

3. Be a good friend and have good friends.
Can friends help each other be healthy?

4. Show care and concern for others.
How does helping others help you?

5. Find ways to deal with stress.
How does this keep you healthy?

6. Think before you speak.
How could this change your communication with others?

7. Think before you act.
What effect would this have on the way you make choices?

8. Choose the positive over the negative.
How would believing things can work out for the best affect your life?

9. Ask yourself how your choices affect others.
How would this influence your relationships with family and friends?

10. Ask for help when you need it.
How do you know when it's time to do this?

Are there any other life lessons you would add to this list?

© ETR

Looking at My Emotional Health

Directions: Use the following prompts to write what you know or think about bullying—whether you have seen it, done it, or watched it happen to others. You will not have to share what you write on this page unless you want to.

1. List at least 5 traits or qualities of good emotional health. Then put a star by the ones you think you already have.

   _____

   _____

   _____

2. How do these qualities help a person be healthy?

   _____

   _____

   _____

   _____

   _____

3. Name a role model you know who has good emotional health. Give an example of a trait of good emotional health that this person has that you admire.

   _____

   _____

   _____

   _____

   _____

   _____

© ETR

My Healthy Relationships

Think about a healthy relationship you have with someone in your family.

• What are 2 qualities of this family relationship?

_____

_____

• What is 1 good thing you get from this family relationship?

_____

Think about a healthy relationship you have with someone your own age.

• What are 2 qualities of this friendship?

_____

_____

• What is 1 good thing you get from this friendship?

_____

_____

• Why is it important to share your feelings in a healthy relationship?

_____

_____

_____

• Why is it also important to try to understand the other person's feelings?

_____

_____

_____

_____

© ETR

Communicating in Winning Ways

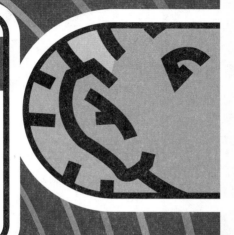

People and relationships are an important part of our lives. They make our days more interesting and more fun. It's great to have someone to talk to about everyday things. It's also great to have someone to talk to when you have problems or need good advice.

Keeping a good relationship going takes time and work. How well you listen to others and communicate your own wants, needs and feelings can help or hurt your relationships.

These ideas can help:

- ◎ Treat others with respect. Use words that show respect.
- ◎ Be sure your body language shows respect too.
- ◎ Use clear language to share your thoughts and feelings.
- ◎ Calm down before you express strong feelings.
- ◎ Choose a good time to talk with others or ask your questions.
- ◎ Think before you speak. Share how you feel, then *listen*. Give the other person a chance to speak.
- ◎ Find the courage to talk about and get help for problems.
- ◎ Learn from your relationships and experiences.

Think about your communication skills:

What are you getting better at?

What still needs work?

Getting Good Health Information

Good health is important! You already know and do things to be and stay healthy. But where do you go when you have questions about your health?

People and places that we go to for help are also called resources.

You want to be sure the resources you use to answer questions about health are accurate. This means the information or advice they provide is based on proven facts and not just made up.

You also want to find resources that are reliable. This means you can count on them to give you correct information and tell you the truth.

There are lots of different resources:

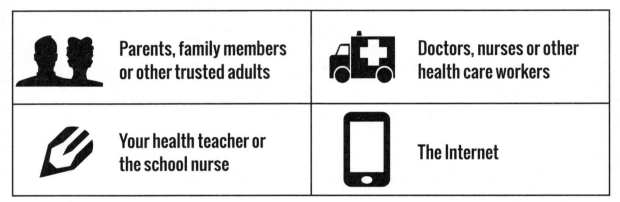

Parents, family members or other trusted adults	Doctors, nurses or other health care workers
Your health teacher or the school nurse	The Internet

There is a lot of great information about health available online. But you also need to be careful when you search. **Here's why:**

- Some people or private businesses use the Internet as an easy and quick way to reach people with ideas, advice, products and services they believe in or want to sell to make money.
- Some online health information is false or wrong.
- Some products or services don't really work or have never been tested by scientists or agreed on by experts to be safe or healthy.

It's important to learn how to assess a health website to decide if you can trust the information, services or products you find there.

© ETR

5 Questions
to Ask About a
Health Website

? Who made the website? Was the website created by an individual person or company (.com), a government agency (.gov), a college or other school (.edu), or a nonprofit organization (.org)? Websites that end in .gov, .org or .edu are likely to be more reliable than commercial or private websites.

? What's the website's point of view? Is it based on one person's opinion, or is it backed up by facts? Is there data from studies or statements from experts? Are there links to and from these sources?

? When was the website created or updated? Most reliable websites will state when the information was posted. Is the date easy to find? Do the links on the website still work?

? Whom is the website for? Is the information meant for kids? teens? adults? experts? people who work in health care? everyone?

? Is the website trying to get you to buy, do or believe something? Does it play on your feelings or use words meant to persuade people? Sometimes companies or people who want to sell a product will stretch the truth or make claims that aren't backed up by facts.

These questions can help you decide if you've found a reliable website that can give you accurate and useful information. These same questions can help you assess other resources too, such as books, pamphlets, magazines, and radio or TV shows.

Where Would You Go?

Directions: List a person or place you could go to for answers or advice in the following situations. Explain why you would choose this resource and how you know it is reliable.

If you want to know...	You can get help or advice from...
What is the best way to get fit?	
Am I getting sick?	
How much sleep do I need each night?	
Why do I feel this way?	
How can I get someone to like me?	

© ETR

Common Chronic Diseases

Heart Disease

What is does: Your heart is the organ that pumps blood to all the different parts of your body through a network of blood vessels.

For more information, you can visit these websites:

http://kidshealth.org/en/kids/heart-disease.html
https://www.cdc.gov/heartdisease/

The blood gives your cells the oxygen they need to function and stay healthy. When there are problems with the heart or blood vessels a person has heart disease. Some forms of heart disease affect the blood vessels while others affect the heart itself. A heart attack can occur when a blood clot or other blockage cuts off the blood flow to the heart.

How to prevent it: Smoking, high blood pressure, being overweight and not getting enough physical activity can all increase a person's risk for heart disease. You can reduce your risk by staying tobacco free, eating healthy foods, being at a healthy weight and being physically active every day.

Stroke

What it does: A stroke happens when something stops the normal flow of blood to a person's brain. This can happen when a blood

For more information, you can visit these websites:

http://kidshealth.org/en/kids/stroke.html
https://www.cdc.gov/stroke/

vessel gets blocked or even bursts. When a person has a stroke, brain cells die or are damaged because they don't get the oxygen they need. A stroke can cause one side of the body to become numb or weak. It can affect the person's ability to talk, walk or do everyday things.

How to prevent it: Many of the same things that help prevent heart disease also help prevent strokes. Smoking, drinking too much alcohol, high blood pressure, and not getting enough physical activity can all increase a person's risk. You can reduce your risk by staying tobacco and alcohol free, eating healthy foods and being physically active every day.

(continued)

© ETR

Cancer

For more information, you can visit these websites:

http://kidshealth.org/en/kids/cancer-center/cancer-basics
https://www.cdc.gov/cancer

What it does: Cancer happens when certain cells in the body begin to divide without stopping and spread very fast. It can happen in many different parts of the body. Often the cancer cells form a lump or a group of cells called a tumor. The tumor can destroy the normal body cells around it and cause damage. Cancer cells can also break away and travel to other parts of the body where they form new tumors. Most of the time, cancers affect older people. But kids can get certain forms of cancer too. There are more than 100 kinds of cancer.

How to prevent it: People can't always prevent cancer. It can happen due to a person's genes or things in the environment. But making healthy choices can help reduce your risk. Don't smoke and avoid being around other people's tobacco smoke. Protect your skin from the sun. Stay at a healthy weight by eating healthy and being physically active. And avoid drinking too much alcohol as an adult. It's also important for people to get tested or screened for certain kinds of cancer, especially if someone else in their family has had it.

Diabetes

For more information, you can visit these websites:

http://kidshealth.org/en/kids/type2.html
https://www.cdc.gov/diabetes/basics/diabetes.html

What it does: Diabetes is a disease that affects how the body uses something called glucose. Glucose is a type of sugar that is the body's main source of energy. Your body gets glucose from the food you eat. A hormone called insulin helps move this glucose into the body's cells. When a person has diabetes, the glucose isn't able to get from the bloodstream into the cells. Then the amount of sugar in the blood gets too high and can make the person sick.

There are two types of diabetes. With Type 1, the body doesn't make insulin to help move the glucose into the cells. With Type 2 diabetes, the body makes insulin, but the insulin doesn't work well. Type 2 diabetes is the kind that you can help prevent by making healthy choices.

How to prevent it: The tendency to get diabetes can be passed down through families. But one big risk factor for type 2 diabetes is being overweight. Stay at a healthy weight by eating healthy and being physically active every day. Research has shown that regular physical activity can reduce the risk of type 2 diabetes in a big way.

© ETR

My Lifestyle and My Future

Directions: Read and think about whether you do each of these things.
Circle **Never**, **Sometimes** or **Every Day** for each one. Then answer the questions.

1. I eat a variety of fruits and vegetables.   **Never**   **Sometimes**   **Every Day**

2. I exercise.   **Never**   **Sometimes**   **Every Day**

3. I choose to be tobacco free.   **Never**   **Sometimes**   **Every Day**

4. I stay away from secondhand smoke.   **Never**   **Sometimes**   **Every Day**

5. I drink plenty of water.   **Never**   **Sometimes**   **Every Day**

6. I choose to be alcohol free.   **Never**   **Sometimes**   **Every Day**

7. I wash my hands often during the day.   **Never**   **Sometimes**   **Every Day**

8. I wash my hands when I am around
people who are sick.   **Never**   **Sometimes**   **Every Day**

Questions

1. What does this survey tell you about your health choices?
(Circle your answer.)

    A. My lifestyle choices need a lot of work!

    B. My lifestyle choices are OK, but could be better.

    C. My lifestyle choices are predicting a healthy future for me!

(continued)

My Lifestyle and My Future

(continued)

2. What things will you keep on doing to be healthy?

_____

_____

_____

3. What kinds of things will you start doing or do better to be healthy?

_____

_____

_____

4. Why is a healthy lifestyle important to you?

_____

_____

_____

_____

_____

_____

_____

_____

_____

Speed Write: What Bullying Means to Me

Directions: Use the following prompts to write what you think, feel and know about bullying—whether you have seen it, done it, or watched it happen to others. You will not have to share what you write unless you want to.

1. When I hear the word *bullying*, I think...

_____

_____

_____

_____

_____

2. When I hear the word *bullying*, I feel...

_____

_____

_____

_____

_____

3. When I hear the word *bullying*, I know...

_____

_____

_____

_____

_____

© ETR

STORIES ABOUT BULLYING

Kieren

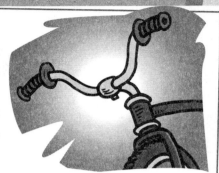

When I was in fifth grade there was this boy in my neighborhood who bullied me all the time. He was a year older, in sixth grade. I put up with his name calling and teasing for a long time. But it got worse.

One day when I was riding my bike I saw him standing in front of his house with some other kids. As I rode by, he ran over, grabbed the handlebars, and knocked me off my bike. His friends all laughed.

Marcus

When I started sixth grade I was really small. There was this kid, an eighth grader, who I used to see in the hallway sometimes during the passing period. He was huge, maybe 6 feet tall.

One day I was minding my own business, just walking to class. I tried to walk behind him, and he leaned back and pinned me against the wall with his backpack! He leaned with all his weight so I couldn't move. He acted as if I wasn't there—he just kept talking to his friends.

Emily

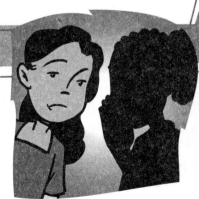

When I was in the fifth grade my family moved and I started going to a new school. One day my mom and dad picked me up after school. The next day, this girl in my class asked if they were my parents. I said, "Yes, of course they're my parents." She said they couldn't be my parents because we didn't look the same. Well, she was right about that. I was born in Korea. My parents adopted me when I was a baby.

Every day after that, this girl would say things like my real mom didn't love me or she would never have given me away. She and her friends would whisper mean things to me whenever I walked past them. I started to hate going to school.

Then it got even worse. One day when I got on my computer, I saw that this girl had started posting mean things online about me being adopted. I know a lot of people at school saw what she wrote. I hadn't told my parents what was going on because I didn't want them to feel bad, and now I was afraid to tell them in case they wouldn't let me go online any more.

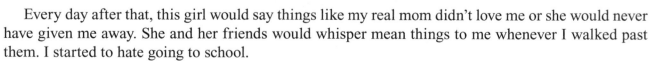

© ETR

Why Kids Bully

John

John's family has just moved and he is the "new kid" at a new school. John feels out of place and misses his old friends. He spent his first recess wandering around the playground by himself. As the kids were lining up outside the classroom after recess, John cut in line by stepping in front of a much smaller kid named Ivan.

When Ivan began to complain, John flipped Ivan's baseball cap off his head. When Ivan bent over to pick up his hat, John kicked the hat out of his reach. Some of the other boys in line were laughing.

Layla

Layla has trouble keeping her grades up in school. No matter how hard she tries, she always seems to make bad grades. Her parents were very disappointed with her last report card. Layla started to give Annette, one of the top students in the class, a hard time.

She began by teasing Annette, calling her names like "nerd" and "brainiac" when the teacher can't hear. She makes fun of the clothes Annette wears, and how she looks. At lunch, when Annette tries to talk to Layla, Layla ignores her.

The Girls' Club

Laura, Josie and Shantay have known each other since the first grade. They became really close friends when they were all in the same fifth grade class. They felt that some of the other girls in the class got more attention than they did, so they decided to start their own "Girls' Club" with a membership of three.

One of their favorite things to do is to start rumors about other kids in the class. They especially like to pick on a girl named Amy, who is quiet and shy. No one knows Amy very well, so it is easy to start rumors. They passed mean notes to other kids in the class, and posted comments on some classmates's social media pages signed by "Amy." Amy didn't understand why everyone seemed to be angry with her.

Simon

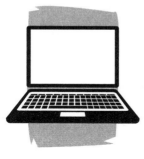

Simon is known at school as someone who stays out of trouble and follows the rules. But Simon has a secret—he is a cyberbully. Simon likes the power he has with his computer. He says things online that he would never say in person. It all started when he saw a mean comment online about a girl at his school and passed it on to some of his friends. When his friends thought it was funny and liked it, Simon felt cool. He started making up his own mean messages and posting them on people's pages and the school's website.

Speed Write Take 2:
What Bullying Means to Me Now

The difference between bullying and teasing is...

_____

_____

_____

_____

_____

Some reasons people might bully others are...

_____

_____

_____

_____

_____

It is wrong to bully others because of how they look, act or dress because...

_____

_____

_____

_____

_____

_____

© ETR

Bullying & CYBERBULLYING

Many people—adults, teens and people your age—could tell you a story about a problem they've had with a bully. Bullying can happen in many ways.

BULLYING is when one person hurts another on purpose and more than once. Whenever people use their power to hurt, make fun of or reject someone else, and do this more than once, they are bullying.

Bullies use their power in many ways. They call names. They threaten. They steal or damage other people's belongings. They spread rumors. They write mean things. They use physical abuse such as punching, kicking and pushing. They try to make other people do things they don't want to do.

CYBERBULLYING is when a bully goes online or uses any kind of technology to hurt other people. Cyberbullies can't hurt someone physically, but they can still do a lot of harm. They can start rumors or post cruel or embarrassing things. Cyberbullying can even be meaner than face-to-face bullying, because once something is online, it never goes away.

With cyberbullying, the bully can target someone 24 hours a day, any day of the week. Cyberbullies can be extra mean because they don't have to face the people they are hurting.

Have you ever been a bully or a cyberbully?

Have you ever been a target of bullying or cyberbullying?

Have you ever been a bystander to bullying or cyberbullying?

BYSTANDERS are the people who watch or know about someone being bullied. They might see the bully hurt someone. They might hear about the bullying from someone else. They might read or even pass on mean comments someone posted about someone else online. Bystanders have a role to play in bullying. They can ignore it or pretend it isn't happening. They can join in and make the bullying worse. Or they can stand up for the person who is being bullied and help take steps to stop it.

© ETR

Bullying & Feelings

Here is a list of how bullying can make people feel:

helpless

ASHAMED

frustrated

angry

lonely

sad

isolated

depressed

humiliated

embarrassed

inferior

overwhelmed

intimidated

worthless

© ETR

Bullying: What Could Happen?

Directions: Choose one of the **Stories About Bullying** on page 14. Then write what could have happened next for each of the people involved.

_____'s Story: What Happened Next

Who was the target of the bullying? (circle the name of the person whose story you chose)

Kieren   **Marcus**   **Emily**

How did this person feel because of the bullying?

_____

What else could happen to this person because of the bullying?

_____

_____

Who were the bystanders who knew about the bullying?

_____

How did the bystanders feel because of the bullying?

_____

_____

What else could happen to the bystanders because of the bullying?

_____

_____

Who was doing the bullying? _____

What could happen to the bully?

_____

_____

_____

Bullying Story Ending 1

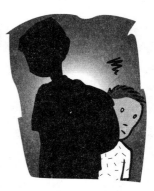

Directions: Read the ending to the story. As a group, write down what you think the good and bad outcomes could be from this story ending. Be prepared to share your answers.

Ending 1

When the eighth grader let him go, Marcus decided to ignore the situation and walk away. He didn't tell any classmates or adults about what happened.

Positive outcomes from this decision:

_____

_____

_____

_____

_____

_____

_____

_____

_____

_____

_____

_____

Negative outcomes from this decision:

_____

_____

_____

_____

_____

_____

_____

_____

_____

_____

_____

_____

Bullying Story Ending 2

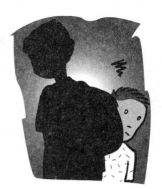

Directions: Read the ending to the story. As a group, write down what you think the good and bad outcomes could be from this story ending. Be prepared to share your answers.

Ending 2

Marcus decided to stand up tall, look the bully straight in the eye and say in a strong voice, "Leave me alone."

Positive outcomes from this decision:	Negative outcomes from this decision:
_____	_____
_____	_____
_____	_____
_____	_____
_____	_____
_____	_____
_____	_____
_____	_____
_____	_____
_____	_____
_____	_____
_____	_____
_____	_____
_____	_____

© ETR

Bullying Story Ending 3

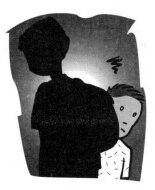

Directions: Read the ending to the story. As a group, write down what you think the good and bad outcomes could be from this story ending. Be prepared to share your answers.

Ending 3

Marcus decided to go tell a teacher about what the eighth grader had done to him. The teacher didn't believe him, so he went and told the school counselor.

Positive outcomes from this decision:	Negative outcomes from this decision:
_____	_____
_____	_____
_____	_____
_____	_____
_____	_____
_____	_____
_____	_____
_____	_____
_____	_____
_____	_____
_____	_____
_____	_____
_____	_____

© ETR

Breaking the "No Tell Code"

Directions: Read the story and answer the questions.

You are in the hallway on your way to class and see Marcus being bullied. A big eighth grader is talking to some friends. When Marcus tries to walk behind him, the eighth grader leans back and pins Marcus against the wall with his backpack. It looks like it hurts, and you can tell that Marcus is upset. The eighth grader and his friends just keep talking and pretend not to notice what's happening to Marcus.

What would you do?

_____

_____

_____

_____

What other things can bystanders do to help prevent or stop bullying?

_____

_____

_____

_____

Write what you would say to a friend to explain how breaking the "No Tell Code" can help prevent bullying.

_____

_____

_____

_____

Fights: Pieces of the Puzzle

Directions: Fill in your ideas in each section.

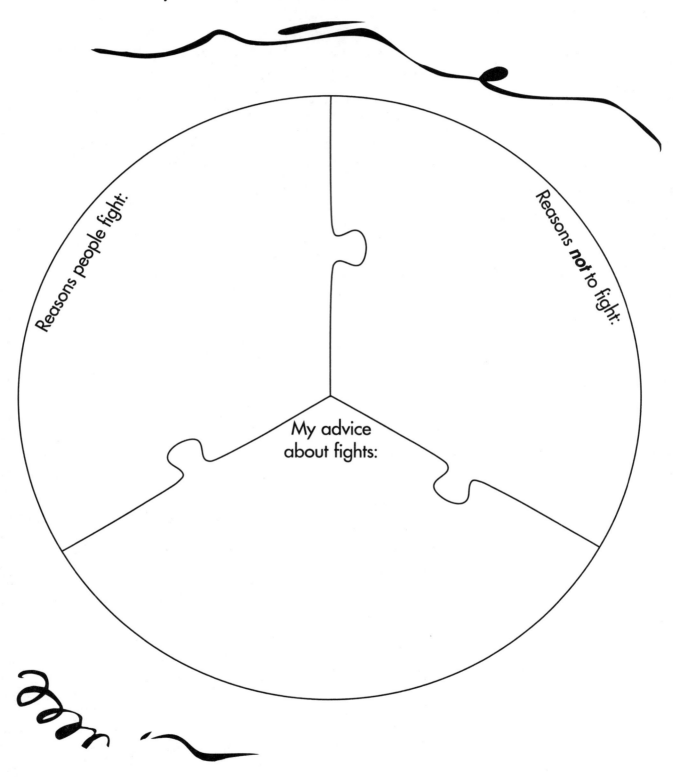

Reasons people fight:

Reasons **not** to fight:

My advice about fights:

Top 6 Reasons for Fights

1. People lose their tempers. One minute a group is playing basketball, the next minute two of them are fighting. It usually starts as an argument: "You fouled me!" "I did not!" Words can lead to pushing and shoving, which can lead to a serious fight.

2. Dares and peer pressure. Sometimes people may think they have to fight. If they don't, friends will call them names or will say they "chickened out." Some people like to start fights themselves. Some use peer pressure to start fights between others.

3. Jealousy. Fights can happen because one person is jealous of another, or when two people like the same boy or girl. Some times people are jealous of others because of the way they dress, the amount of attention they get, or because they do well in school and sports.

4. Rumors and gossip. Spreading rumors and gossiping often starts fights. People get angry when untrue things are said about them. When they don't know how to peacefully solve conflict, they fight with those they think are spreading the rumors.

5. Gangs. Fighting is often expected of the members of a gang. Gangs may fight with other gangs for power or territory. They may make anyone who wants to join the gang fight or commit other acts of violence.

6. Thrill seeking. Some people just like the feeling of danger. Fighting is a risky behavior and they like the thrill that comes from it. They don't think about the serious consequences.

© ETR

Top 10 Reasons Not to Fight

1. School fights can be dangerous.

2. There is a chance weapons can be involved.

3. You can seriously hurt someone.

4. You can get seriously hurt.

5. One fight often sets off another fight.

6. You can lose friends.

7. Fights don't solve problems—you may have to fight again and again.

8. You can get in trouble and be suspended from school.

9. You can get arrested for assault.

10. Your parents can get sued if you hurt someone.

Fights: Putting the Puzzle Together

Directions: Use what you've learned about fights to answer the questions.

What are 3 reasons people might fight?

1. _____

2. _____

3. _____

Name 3 good reasons not to fight.

1. _____

2. _____

3. _____

How could being in gang increase a person's chance of being in a fight?

_____

_____

_____

_____

_____

_____

_____

_____

_____

_____

© ETR

Fights & Feelings

JEFF'S DAY
STARTED OUT BADLY AND GOT WORSE.

His mom left him a note reminding him to unload the dishwasher and take out the trash before he left for school. The trash bag broke on the way to the yard and there was a big mess to clean up. Now Jeff was running late for school. He jumped on his bike and raced off.

Jeff made it to school only to discover that he'd forgotten to put his homework in his backpack. He'd stayed up late to work on it and now he'd get a zero because his teacher didn't accept late assignments.

Jeff tried to concentrate on the math lesson, but it wasn't making sense. Then his teacher announced a quiz for the next day and assigned 30 practice problems. Jeff thought, "Great! And I've got baseball practice tonight. How am I going to get all of this done?" The day was turning into a real stress-fest.

During lunch break Jeff joined in a basketball game. It was fun at first. It helped take Jeff's mind off his miserable morning. This guy named Daryl started to foul Jeff whenever Jeff had the ball. The fouling started to get really rough and that's when Jeff finally lost it. He shoved Daryl hard, Daryl shoved back, and two seconds later they were fighting. Other kids quickly gathered around them, chanting, "Fight! Fight!"

Teachers pushed through the crowd and separated the two boys. Jeff looked down at his shirt and saw that it was bloody. His nose was bleeding, and Daryl's eye was swelling up. As the boys were marched off to the principal's office, Jeff was feeling very scared about what his mom was going to say. Daryl looked like he was scared too.

After the Fight

Directions: Write an ending to the **Fights & Feelings** story. In your ending, be sure to include at least three things that happened to Jeff and/or Daryl because of the fight. Include something about feelings they had and the consequences they faced at school and at home. Then answer the questions at the bottom of the page.

After the fight...

Questions:

What are some ways people try to make others fight?

_____

_____

_____

_____

_____

What influence do you think your peers have on fights here at school?

_____

_____

_____

_____

_____

© ETR

The Soccer Conflict

Alex and CJ have been friends since third grade. But lately they haven't spent as much time with each other. They are both feeling a little sad about this, but haven't talked about it with each other.

Today at recess they were playing soccer with some classmates. Alex kicked the ball hard and it hit CJ in the back. When the other kids laughed, CJ got mad. CJ yelled at Alex, "You did that on purpose!" This wasn't true, but Alex yelled back, "So what if I did! What are you going to do about it?" CJ ran up and shoved Alex, and Alex shoved CJ back. The other kids stopped laughing and everyone was watching Alex and CJ.

What do you think happened next?

What could have helped Alex and CJ not get into a fight?

What could the bystanders do to help Alex and CJ avoid fighting?

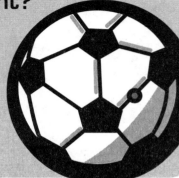

© ETR

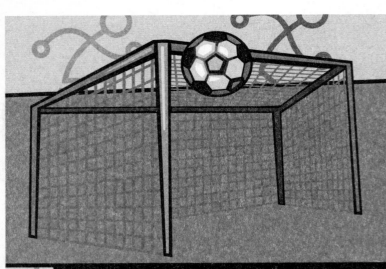

SIMPLE CONFLICT OR SERIOUS TROUBLE?

ENDING 1

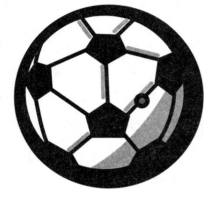

After they shoved each other, Alex and CJ both took a deep breath. They just stood there looking at each other. Then CJ started to laugh. Alex was surprised, but then started smiling too. Alex said, "I really wasn't aiming for you." CJ said, "I know. Let's keep playing."

Was this a simple conflict or serious trouble?

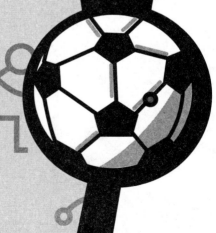

ENDING 2

Alex and CJ kept shoving each other. A teacher noticed and came over to break up the fight. But when the teacher left, CJ whispered to Alex, "Just wait. I'll get you after school!"

Was this a simple conflict or the start of serious trouble?

© ETR

When Friends or Classmates

Need Help

Violence at school is something we can all live *without*. But, it seems that every few months there's another story about a tragic school event. Most of us will never experience these kinds of tragedies. But is there anything we can do to make our schools safer?

Yes. You can learn to notice warning signs that tell you a friend or classmate may need help.

Here are some early warning signs:

- Threatening to hurt oneself or other people
- An interest in weapons, bombs and violence, and in movies, music, computer games, etc., that highlight these things
- Drinking alcohol or using other drugs

- Displays of anger that is out of control
- Withdrawal from friends and activities
- Having no friends

- Having been a victim of violence
- Expressing a desire for revenge
- Feeling picked on or persecuted
- Hurting animals

- Threatening suicide
- Writing stories about violence, or drawing pictures of violent acts
- An interest in gangs or being in a gang

- Getting bad grades, losing interest in school
- Being a "troublemaker" at school or elsewhere
- Not going to class or skipping school often

If you see these warning signs in a friend or classmate, get help before there is a crisis. Talk to an adult you can trust.

© ETR

Helping a Friend: What Can You Do?

Directions: Read the stories and answer the questions.

Katya

Katya has been having a really hard time lately. Some girls in her class have been posting mean comments on her social media page and have been spreading rumors about her at school. Katya feels too embarrassed about what's being said to tell her parents about the bullying. She is avoiding everyone and feeling hopeless and depressed. Last night when she went online, someone had posted a message saying that the world would be a better place if Katya wasn't in it and that nobody would miss her if she was gone. Katya sat silently crying in front of her computer for a very long time.

What are the warning signs that Katya needs help?

_____

_____

_____

What might happen if Katya doesn't get help?

_____

_____

_____

What could you say or do to help Katya?

_____

_____

_____

Why is it important to ask an adult for help in this situation?

_____

_____

_____

(continued)

© ETR

Helping a Friend: What Can You Do?

(continued)

James

James is a friend of yours. But lately you've almost been afraid to talk to him. He seems angry all the time and is always arguing with you and his other friends. Yesterday he almost got suspended for starting a fight. You tried to talk to him about it after school, but he yelled, "Leave me alone!" and walked away.

What are the warning signs that James needs help?

_____

_____

_____

What might happen if James doesn't get help?

_____

_____

_____

What would you say or do to help James?

_____

_____

_____

Why is it important to ask an adult for help in this situation?

_____

_____

_____

MEDIA VIOLENCE & YOU

Television, movies, music videos, magazines and the Internet are all types of media that have the power to entertain us, inform us and educate us. But some elements of the media also have the power to influence us.

What you choose to eat, or to wear, or what shows and movies you like to watch is often based on what you see and hear in the media. Advertisers use the media to sell you on their products. They understand so much about the power of the media that they spend millions of dollars each year on messages for kids like you!

Not convinced? Check out the clothes you and your friends are wearing. What brand names do you see? How many soft drinks can you name? How do you decide what movies you want to see? What's your favorite commercial?

Many people believe that TV shows, movies and video games also have the power to influence the way you think, act, and feel—and the way you make choices about what is important.

When people see yelling, screaming, name calling, shoving, hitting, kicking, stabbing and shooting in the media, and this happens over and over again, some tend to believe that violence is normal—and that it is acceptable. What do you think? Do you have evidence for your opinion?

* **What's the important idea or message about the media and violence?**

* **What's this got to do with you or the people you care about?**

It's Casual, It's Cruel

It's Casual Cruelty

Your favorite TV show or Internet video may be really funny, but life is not a sitcom. TV shows often use put-downs, name calling and disrespect to get laughs. They show characters based on stereotype—a set idea of how an individual or a group of people "should" look or act. Often based on ethnic, cultural or physical qualities, these stereotypes are used as humor. But what seems funny on TV or online can be very different when the same thing happens to us in real life.

Stereotyping, name calling and put-downs are all examples of behavior called "casual cruelty." We could carelessly say or do something disrespectful or even harmful and think it's funny or OK because we see it and hear it all the time on TV or online. But casual cruelty becomes a bad habit, something we do without even thinking about it.

To break the casual cruelty habit, we have to start by *noticing* when it happens. *Notice* where a comment or action that feels OK may actually hurt or upset someone else.

What examples of casual cruelty have you seen lately in the media (TV, movies, Internet, video games)?

© ETR

Casual Cruelty in the Media

Directions: Watch a TV show or some Internet videos tonight. Make a tally each time a character does any of these things. Then answer the question.

Action	Tally
Calls someone a name	
Insults or puts down another character	
Uses a stereotype	
Treats someone with disrespect	

What is the message?

_____

_____

_____

Is this message true? Why or why not?

_____

_____

_____

If people believe the message, what could happen?

_____

_____

_____

© ETR

HealthSmart Guidelines for Healthy Eating

Eat a Variety of Foods in Healthy Amounts

Has your eating become predictable? Have you gotten into a "food-choice rut"?

Variety means mix it up—choose different foods to meet your nutritional needs. Cereal and milk is a good breakfast choice. Slice a banana or peach onto the cereal or grab a glass of fruit juice to be sure you get some fruit early in the day. Or how about a fruit smoothie made with fruit, low-fat yogurt and milk?

For lunch, have sandwiches with different fillings on different types of bread. Or try soups, salads, a baked potato with healthy toppings or a bean burrito instead of a sandwich. Add carrot or celery sticks and a piece of fruit.

Eat a Variety of Whole-Grain Foods Daily

Whole-grain foods come in many delicious forms: whole-wheat cinnamon raisin bread, pasta salad with fresh veggies, oatmeal, a warm corn tortilla, a steaming bowl of brown rice, or whole-wheat pita bread stuffed with a tasty filling. These are the foods that provide the energy your body needs, especially when you're going through a growth spurt or are physically active.

Kids should eat about 5 to 8 ounces of grains a day. At least half the grains should be whole grains.

Here are some examples. All of these equal 1 ounce of grains:
- 1 cup of cold cereal—you're probably pouring 2 or 3 cups into your bowl, which gives you 2 to 3 ounces at breakfast.
- 1 slice of bread—so a sandwich for lunch gives you 2 ounces.
- ½ cup of cooked rice or pasta, or about 32 strands of spaghetti— you probably eat a cup, or 2 ounces, at dinner.

So it's not hard at all to get 5 to 8 ounces in a day. Remember that whole grains are better, so try to eat whole-wheat instead of white bread. And cereals are great, but avoid the sugary ones.

Eat a Variety of Fruits and Vegetables Daily

The good news is that you can eat lots of fruits and vegetables. The bad news is that you're probably not eating nearly enough to be really healthy. Each day you should be eating 1½ to 3 cups of veggies and 1½ to 2 cups of fruit.

Here are some examples:
- ½ cup of raw or cooked vegetables such as carrots, bell peppers, broccoli or corn.
- 2 cups of raw leafy vegetables such as spinach or lettuce equal 1 cup of vegetables.
- 1 small apple, orange or banana equals ½ cup of fruit.

It's important to eat a variety of fruits and vegetables. Vegetables supply your body with vitamins you may not get from other foods. Fruits are your best source of vitamin C and also supply carbohydrates for quick energy. Fruits and vegetables also give you fiber to keep your digestive system healthy.

(continued)

© ETR

It's not hard to add fruits and vegetables to your routine. Stick a piece of fruit in your backpack to eat when you need a power surge. Try kiwis, nectarines, dried cranberries or pears. Instead of a soft drink, have a glass of orange or cranberry juice. Slice up some crisp bell peppers or pack a small bag of baby carrots for lunch or a snack. Adding fruits and veggies to your food plan is easy, fun and healthy.

Eat a Variety of Lean Protein Foods

Protein is an important building block for healthy bones, muscles, skin and blood. These foods also give your body vitamins and minerals. You should have 5 to 6½ ounces of protein foods each day.

Here are some examples. All of these equal 1 ounce:

- 1 ounce of cooked fish, lean beef, pork or ham
- 1 ounce cooked chicken or turkey without the skin
- 1 egg
- ½ ounce of nuts (12 almonds, 24 pistachios, 7 walnut halves)
- 1 tablespoon of peanut butter
- ¼ cup cooked beans or peas
- ¼ cup tofu

Most people in the United States eat enough protein already.

Eat Low-Fat Dairy Foods Daily

Dairy foods include milk, cheese and yogurt. These foods keep your bones and teeth healthy and help build muscles. You need 2 to 3 cups each day. If you stick with low-fat dairy foods you get vitamin D, calcium and protein without added fat and calories. Try making kabobs by alternating low-fat cheese and fruit chunks on a toothpick (6 small chunks of cheese equals 1 cup of milk). It's easy to grab a container of low-fat yogurt, or choose a glass of low-fat milk with a meal. (One cup of milk is 8 ounces, the size of the small carton you get at school.)

Eat Less Sugar, Fat and Salt

Sugar doesn't give your body nutrients—it just adds calories, and causes tooth decay and cavities. Soft drinks are the number one source of sugar in people's diets. When you're thirsty, try drinking water instead.

Fats are important in small amounts. But milkshakes, burgers, fries and pizza give you way too much of the wrong kind of fat. The fat in many meats and dairy products, called saturated fat, raises blood cholesterol, which isn't good. Choose lean meats and low-fat dairy products. Avoid trans fats, which are found in many processed snack foods.

The fat in vegetable oils, most nuts, and some fish such as salmon and tuna is unsaturated fat. It's a healthier choice than saturated fat.

Salt has been used as a flavoring for thousands of years, but most people consume too much of it. You need only a small amount of salt daily. Most snack foods, canned soups, frozen dinners, ketchup, mustard, soy sauce and pickles contain a lot of salt. Ease up on salty foods and you'll begin to notice and enjoy other food flavors more.

MyPlate

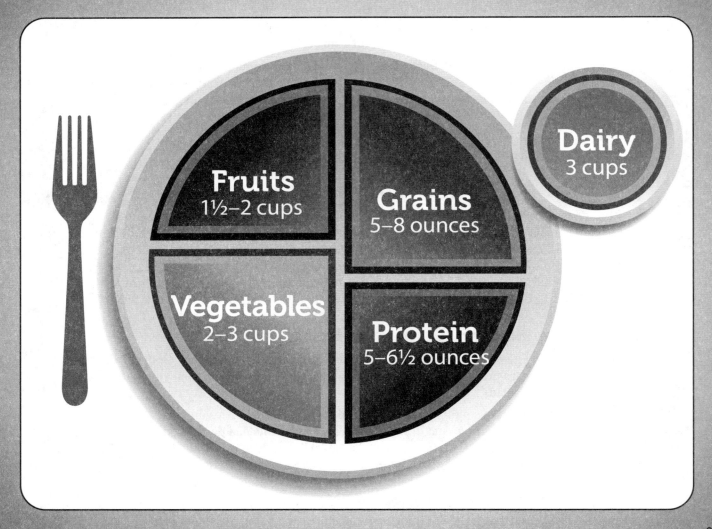

Fruits
1½–2 cups

Grains
5–8 ounces

Vegetables
2–3 cups

Protein
5–6½ ounces

Dairy
3 cups

What's on MyPlate?

Directions: Fill in the names of the food groups and list 2 or 3 healthy foods you like from each group. Then answer the questions.

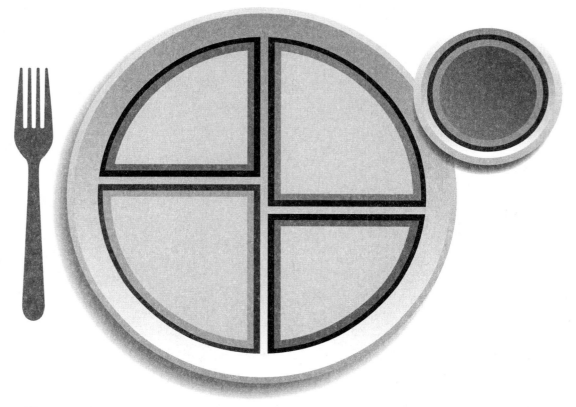

Questions:

Why is it important to eat different foods from all the food groups?

_____

_____

_____

What are the good things you get from eating plenty of fruits and vegetables?

_____

_____

_____

_____

© ETR

How Much Should I Eat?

Grains   You need 5–8 ounces of grains a day.

Each of these equals 1 ounce of grains:

6-inch tortilla

1 slice bread

1/2 hamburger or hot dog bun

1/2 English muffin or 1/2 "mini" bagel

1 small roll, biscuit or muffin

4-inch pita bread

7 saltine crackers

5 whole-wheat crackers

1/2 cup cooked oatmeal

4½ inch pancake

1/2 cup cooked rice

3 rice cakes

12 tortilla chips

1 cup ready-to-eat cereal

1/2 medium donut

3 cups popcorn

3 small cookies

Vegetables   You need 2–3 cups of vegetables a day.

Each of these equals 1/2 cup of vegetables:

1/2 medium baked potato

1/2 cup peas, beans, corn, carrots, cabbage, squash, spinach

1 cup leafy salad or greens

1/2 cup cucumber

1/2 cup broccoli florets

1/2 bell pepper

1 medium chili pepper

1 small ear of corn (6 inches long)

1/2 cup raw or cooked mushrooms

6 baby carrots

1/2 cup coleslaw or potato salad

1/2 cup cooked sweet potato

© ETR

(continued)

How Much Should I Eat? *(continued)*

Fruits **You need 1½–2 cups of fruit a day.**

Each of these equals 1/2 cup of fruit:

1 small orange, apple, pear, peach

16 seedless grapes

4 large strawberries

2 apricots

1/2 cup frozen or canned fruit

1/4 cup dried fruit

1 kiwi

1/2 mango

1/2 medium grapefruit

1/4 papaya

1/8 cantaloupe or honeydew melon

1/2 cup berries

1/2 cup pineapple

4-ounce glass 100% fruit juice

Dairy **You need 3 cups of dairy a day.**

Each of these equals 1 cup of dairy:

8-ounce glass or carton of milk

8-ounce container of yogurt

2 cups cottage cheese

1/2 cup ricotta cheese

1 cup frozen yogurt

1½ ounces cheddar, Monterey Jack or Swiss cheese (2 slices)

3 slices processed cheese

1 cup calcium-fortified soymilk

Protein **You need 5–6½ ounces of protein a day.**

Each of these equals 1 ounce of protein:

1 ounce cooked chicken, turkey, beef, fish, pork

1/4 cup canned tuna, salmon, crab, shrimp

1 ounce ham or bacon

1½ hot dogs

3 thin slices of lunch meat

3 sausage links

1 egg

1/4 cup cooked dried beans

1/2 cup split pea or lentil soup

1 tablespoon peanut butter

1 tablespoon sunflower or pumpkin seeds

1 tablespoon peanuts, walnuts, pecans, piñon nuts

1/4 cup (about 2 ounces) tofu

From Where I Stand: You Are What You Eat

Directions: Circle the answer that best describes your eating habits.

1. **Fruit:** On an average day, how much do you eat? (Do not count fruit juice.)
    A. 1½–2 cups
    B. 1 cup
    C. ½ cup
    D. I don't eat fruit on most days

2. **Grains:** On an average day, how much do you eat (breads, pasta, rice, tortillas and cereal)?
    A. 5–8 ounces
    B. 3–4 ounces
    C. 1–3 ounces
    D. I don't eat any grains most days

3. **Vegetables:** On an average day, how much do you eat?
    A. 2–3 cups
    B. 1–2 cups
    C. ½–1 cup
    D. I don't eat vegetables on most days

4. **Dairy:** On an average day, how much do you have? (Include milk you put on your cereal.)
    A. 3 cups
    B. 2 cups
    C. 1 cup
    D. I don't have dairy on most days

5. **Protein:** On an average day, how much do you have?
    A. 5–6½ ounces
    B. 3–4 ounces
    C. 1–2 ounces
    D. I don't have protein on most days

6. On an average day, how much "junk food" such as candy, chips or soft drinks do you eat?
    A. I don't eat junk food on most days
    B. 1 serving
    C. 2 servings
    D. 3 or more servings

Score yourself. Give yourself:

4 points for each A answer   ___ x 4 = ___

3 points for each B answer   ___ x 3 = ___

2 points for each C answer   ___ x 2 = ___

1 point for each D answer   ___ x 4 = ___

My Total Score is _____

> If you scored 6–12, you've got lots of room for improving your eating!
>
> If you scored 13–19, you still could do more to improve your eating!
>
> If you scored 20 or higher, way to go! Keep up the good work.

Write 2 things you will do to improve your eating.

1. _____

_____

_____

2. _____

_____

_____

© ETR

Making Healthy Food Choices

Directions: Create a list of foods you could eat for each meal and for snacks to get the correct number of servings from each food group. Use the **How Much Should I Eat?** activity sheet and the sample meals as a guide. List the foods and how much you would eat, then add up the amounts from each group.

Sample Breakfast

1 cup cereal	How Many Ounces of Grains? _____1_____
4 large strawberries	How Many Cups of Vegetables? _____0_____
1/2 cup milk	How Many Cups of Fruits? _____1 1/2_____
8-ounce glass orange juice	How Many Cups of Dairy? _____1/2_____
_____	How Many Ounces of Protein? _____0_____

Your Breakfast

_____	How Many Ounces of Grains? _____
_____	How Many Cups of Vegetables? _____
_____	How Many Cups of Fruits? _____
_____	How Many Cups of Dairy? _____
_____	How Many Ounces of Protein? _____

(continued)

© ETR

Making Healthy Food Choices *(continued)*

Sample Lunch

Turkey sandwich: 2 slices of turkey on
whole-wheat bread with 1 slice of cheese
8-ounce carton of milk
12 baby carrots
Small bag of tortilla chips

How Many Ounces of Grains? **3**
How Many Cups of Vegetables? **1**
How Many Cups of Fruits? **0**
How Many Cups of Dairy? **1½**
How Many Ounces of Protein? **2**

Your Lunch

_____
_____
_____
_____
_____

How Many Ounces of Grains? _____
How Many Cups of Vegetables? _____
How Many Cups of Fruits? _____
How Many Cups of Dairy? _____
How Many Ounces of Protein? _____

Sample Dinner

1 small hamburger on
a whole-wheat bun
2 ears of corn
1 cup frozen yogurt
_____

How Many Ounces of Grains? **2**
How Many Cups of Vegetables? **1**
How Many Cups of Fruits? **0**
How Many Cups of Dairy? **1**
How Many Ounces of Protein? **3**

Your Dinner

_____
_____
_____
_____
_____

How Many Ounces of Grains? _____
How Many Cups of Vegetables? _____
How Many Cups of Fruits? _____
How Many Cups of Dairy? _____
How Many Ounces of Protein? _____

© ETR

(continued)

Making Healthy Food Choices *(continued)*

Sample Snacks

1 small apple	How Many Ounces of Grains? ___1___
1 tablespoon peanut butter	How Many Cups of Vegetables? ___0___
2 chocolate chip cookies	How Many Cups of Fruits? ___½___
_____	How Many Cups of Dairy? ___0___
_____	How Many Ounces of Protein? ___1___

Your Snacks

_____	How Many Ounces of Grains? _____
_____	How Many Cups of Vegetables? _____
_____	How Many Cups of Fruits? _____
_____	How Many Cups of Dairy? _____
_____	How Many Ounces of Protein? _____

How Did You Do? Add the total amount for the day from each food group.

Grains—You need 5–8 ounces. How many ounces did you eat? _____

Vegetables—You need 2 to 3 cups. How many cups did you eat? _____

Fruits—You need 1½ to 2 cups. How many cups did you eat? _____

Dairy—You need 3 cups. How many cups did you eat? _____

Protein—You need 5–6½ ounces. How many ounces did you eat? _____

Which food groups did you eat too little of? _____

How can you increase the amount you eat from those food groups? _____

_____

Which food groups did you eat too much of? _____

How can you reduce the amount you eat from those food groups?

_____

_____

Why They Call It Junk Food

You've heard the term "junk food." But have you really thought about what you're eating and drinking when you give into a craving for junk food? Junk foods have very little nutritional value and are often high in calories, fat, salt (sodium) and sugar.

You probably already know that having a candy bar and a soft drink for lunch isn't the best choice. But there may be other junk foods in your diet that you're not as aware of. Check out the nutritional labels on some of your favorite packaged foods. You'll find that many foods—particularly snacks—can contain high amounts of fat, sugar and sodium.

Prepackaged foods such as butter-flavored popcorn, frozen dinners, pizzas, snack puddings, or cookies and chips are also made to be ready to eat and not spoil quickly. So they contain a lot of extra ingredients such as nitrates and artificial coloring and flavors. These ingredients, along with extra sugar, sodium and fat, create what many people call "junk foods."

And while it's true that occasionally eating a handful of chips or a few cookies won't hurt you, if junk food becomes a regular part of your diet, it can start to affect your energy and hurt your health. You won't feel like eating healthy food when you fill up on junk food. And a steady diet of junk food can lead to tooth decay, gaining too much weight, and other future health problems such as heart disease, cancer and diabetes.

Name That Junk Food: Label 1

Nutrition Facts

Serving Size
  1 package (71g)
Calories 280
  Fat Cal. 110

*Percent Daily Values are based on a 2000 calorie diet.

Amount / serving		%DV*			%DV*
Total Fat	12g	18%	**Total Carb.**	41g	14%
Sat. Fat	3g	15%	Dietary Fiber	1g	5%
Cholest.	35mg	11%	Sugars	26g	
Sodium	115mg	5%	**Protein**	3g	

Vitamin A 0% • Vitamin C 0% • Calcium 0% • Iron 8%

Ingredients: Sugar, enriched bleached flour (wheat flour, niacin, reduced iron, thiamin mononitrate [vitamin B1], riboflavin [vitamin B2], folic acid), vegetable shortening (partially hydrogenated soybean and cottonseed oils), chocolate sandwich cookies (sugar, enriched flour [wheat flour, niacin, reduced iron, thiamin mononitrate (vitamin B1), riboflavin (vitamin B2), folic acid], vegetable shortening [partially hydrogenated soybean oil], cocoa [processed with alkali], high fructose corn syrup, corn flour, whey [from milk], cornstarch, baking soda, salt, soy lecithin [emulsifier], vanillin [an artificial flavor], chocolate), eggs, corn syrup, cocoa (processed with alkali), artificial flavor, salt, leavening (baking soda, sodium aluminum phosphate, calcium phosphate), cornstarch.

(continued)

© ETR

Name That Junk Food: Label 2

Nutrition Facts

Serving Size
1 bar
Calories 230
Fat Cal. 130
*Percent Daily Values are based on a 2000 calorie diet.

Amount per serving %DV*

Total Fat	14g	22%	**Total Carb.**	20g	7%
Sat. Fat	4g	35%	Dietary Fiber	1g	4%
Cholest.	5mg	2%	Sugars	18g	
Sodium	35mg	1%	**Protein**	5g	

Vitamin A 0% • Vitamin C 0% • Calcium 8% • Iron 4%

Ingredients: Milk chocolate (milk chocolate contains sugar; milk; cocoa butter; chocolate; soya lecithin, an emulsifier; and vanillin, an artificial flavoring) and almonds.

Name That Junk Food: Label 3

Nutrition Facts
Serving Size: 1 oz.
Servings per Container: 1

Amount per serving

Calories 150   Calories from Fat 90

		%Daily Value
Total Fat	10g	15%
Saturated Fat	3g	15%
Cholesterol	0mg	0%
Sodium	200mg	8%
Total Carbohydrate	15g	5%
Dietary Fiber	1g	4%
Sugars	2g	
Protein	2g	

Vitamin A 0% • Vitamin C 10%
Calcium 0% • Iron 0%
*Percent Daily Values are based on a 2,000 calorie diet.

Ingredients: Potatoes, corn and/or cottonseed oil, salt, sugar, dextrose, maltodextrin, natural flavor, molasses, onion powder, monosodium glutamate, autolyzed yeast, spices, paprika and extractives of paprika, garlic powder, tomato powder, partially hydrogenated (soybean and canola) oils, citric acid, and mesquite smoke flavor.

Name That Junk Food: Label 4

Nutrition Facts
Serving Size: 1 can

Amount per serving

Calories 140

		%Daily Value
Total Fat	0g	0%
Sodium	50mg	2%
Total Carb.	39g	13%
Sugars	39g	
Protein	0g	

*Percent Daily Values are based on a 2,000 calorie diet.

Ingredients: Carbonated water, high fructose corn syrup and/or sucrose, caramel color, phosphoric acid, natural flavors, caffeine.

Answers
Label 1: Snack-food brownie
Label 2: Chocolate bar
Label 3: BBQ potato chips
Label 4: Cola soda

© ETR

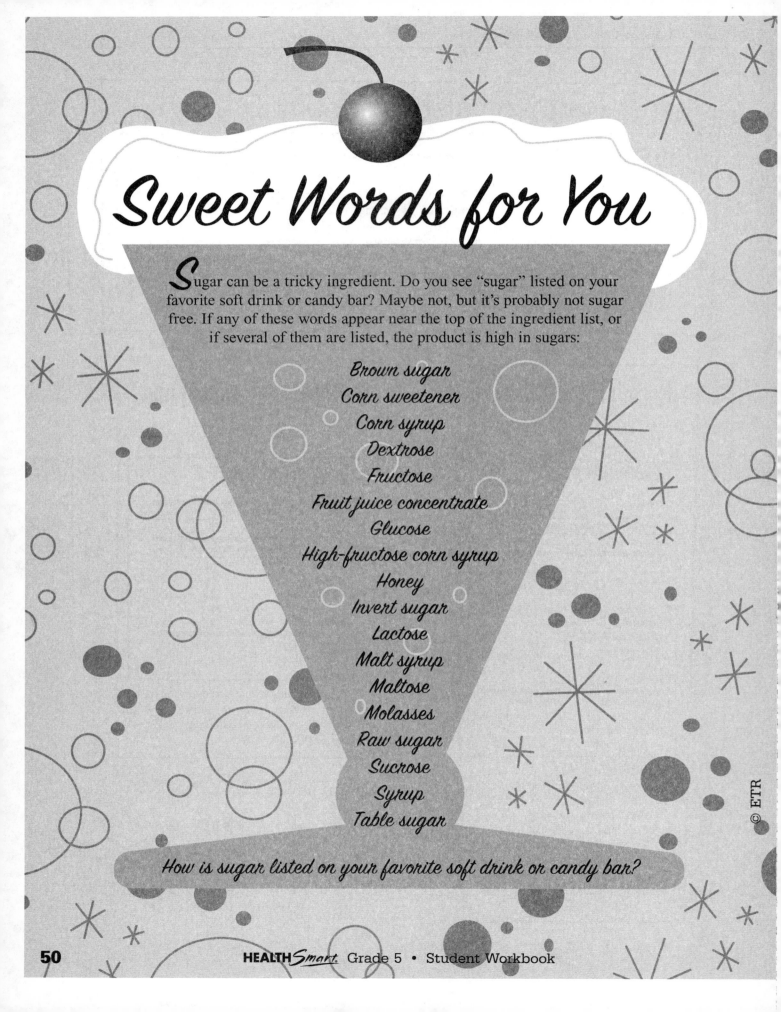

Sweet Words for You

Sugar can be a tricky ingredient. Do you see "sugar" listed on your favorite soft drink or candy bar? Maybe not, but it's probably not sugar free. If any of these words appear near the top of the ingredient list, or if several of them are listed, the product is high in sugars:

Brown sugar
Corn sweetener
Corn syrup
Dextrose
Fructose
Fruit juice concentrate
Glucose
High-fructose corn syrup
Honey
Invert sugar
Lactose
Malt syrup
Maltose
Molasses
Raw sugar
Sucrose
Syrup
Table sugar

How is sugar listed on your favorite soft drink or candy bar?

© ETR

Name _____

Junking the Junk Food

Directions: Fill in the chart with the types of junk food you eat and when you tend to eat these foods. Then write 3 ideas for how you could reduce the amount of junk food you eat and answer the question.

Junk Food	When I Eat It	Is this food...
		☐ High in fat ☐ High in added sugar ☐ High in salt
		☐ High in fat ☐ High in added sugar ☐ High in salt
		☐ High in fat ☐ High in added sugar ☐ High in salt

Questions:

Ways I could limit how much junk food I eat:

_____

_____

_____

_____

What are the good things I will get if I eat less fat, added sugar and salt?

_____

_____

_____

_____

© ETR

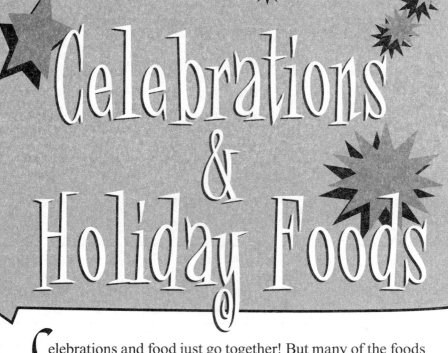

Celebrations & Holiday Foods

Celebrations and food just go together! But many of the foods served on special occasions are high in fat or full of sugar, and people tend to eat too much.

It's easy to think, "Hey, it's a special occasion. It's OK to eat a lot. After all, a holiday like Thanksgiving comes around only once a year." That's true, but if you think about all the celebrations in the year or in your family, and add up all the holidays, birthdays, feast days and other special events, with all the food that goes with them, a person is probably eating a lot of extra calories.

You may be thinking, "So, I've got to give up my birthday cake? No way!" Go ahead and enjoy the birthday cake, but plan how to make the rest of your birthday meal healthier. **Could you:**

- *Snack on veggies instead of chips?*
- *Serve frozen yogurt instead of ice cream?*
- *Have a baked potato or pasta instead of pizza?*
- *Serve fruit juices and sparkling water instead of soda?*

Think about how much you eat on special occasions. Do you really need three helpings of turkey and gravy? Use what you know about healthy serving sizes so you don't overeat.

© ETR

The Fast-Food Challenge

Sometimes it seems as if there's no time to stop and eat. "Fast food" is quick and convenient, especially for busy kids and families. Most teenagers eat up to one-third of their total calories away from home!

One big problem with eating out is the HUGE portions. A regular cheeseburger gives you 3 ounces of meat, 1½ ounces of cheese, 2 ounces of grains, and maybe ½ cup of vegetables if you add lettuce, tomato and onion. A double burger with cheese doubles the amounts. A small order of fries is actually about 2 servings—a "supersize" is almost 4 servings.

It's hard to resist a bargain, and upsizing your fast-food meal for a few cents more can sound like a great deal. But you're buying a lot of stuff your body doesn't need—extra fat, sugar, salt and simply too much of the wrong kind of food. Soft drinks are full of sugar and calories, and special sauces are usually loaded with fat, sugar and salt.

While it won't hurt to eat a fast-food meal once in a while, you should use what you know to eat healthy most of the time. You can learn to plan ahead and develop good "fast-food eating habits."

So how do you look for the healthiest food choices? Here are some ideas:

- *Don't "supersize" your order.*
- *Choose foods that are broiled or grilled, not fried—such as a grilled chicken breast sandwich.*
- *Order a salad.*
- *Get dressings or special sauces on the side. Use only small amounts. Ask for low-fat varieties, if available.*
- *Have a baked potato instead of fries. Try salsa on it instead of butter and sour cream.*

- *Instead of a hamburger, enjoy a sub sandwich with lean meat and lots of veggies such as lettuce, tomato and bell peppers. Ask for mustard instead of mayonnaise, or get the mayo on the side and spread it on lightly.*
- *Get low-fat yogurt with fruit topping instead of ice cream and chocolate sauce for dessert.*
- *Get out of the soft drink habit. Have water, milk or juice instead.*

- *If you do eat a meal with too much fat, sugar or salt, balance it with healthier food the rest of the day and the next. Average food intake over a few days is what counts.*

Even when you're on the run, you can eat food that's good for you!

How Can I Make Fast-Food Meals Healthier?

Directions: Think back to your last meal from a fast-food restaurant or choose a meal from the menu. List the foods you ate. Then plan another fast-food meal with the changes you will make to eat healthier. Don't forget to choose a healthier drink too!

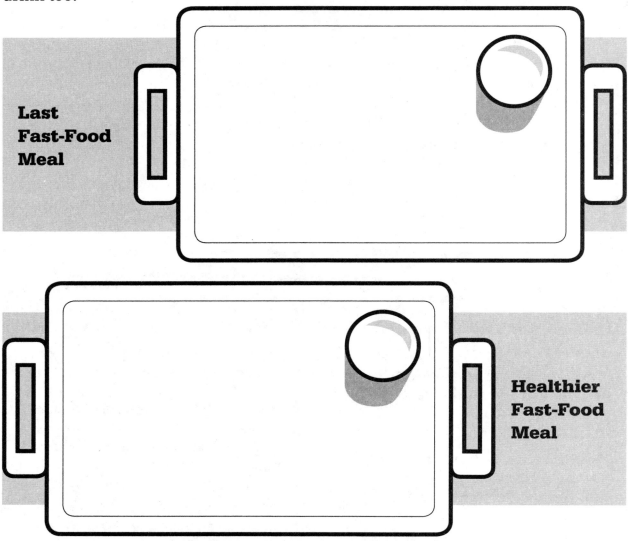

Last Fast-Food Meal

Healthier Fast-Food Meal

© ETR

Things I did to make my meal healthier:

_____

_____

_____

Flexibility, *Endurance* & **Strength**

OK, you've bought into the idea that physical activity and exercise are good things. You're working to get 60 minutes of physical activity each day. Now you may be ready to add another dimension to your fitness—activities that build flexibility, endurance or strength.

Flexibility

Flexibility is the ability to move your jonts freely. It is different than strength. Some people are very strong, but they lack the range of motion that every body needs. You can easily develop flexibility by taking a few minutes each day to stretch your body. You don't have to be a dancer or gymnast. Yoga, tai chi, karate and dancing all include stretching and build flexibility, and have the added benefit of being relaxing and good stress busters.

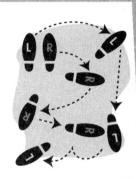

Endurance

Building the endurance that strengthens the entire body, including the heart and lungs, is easy—it just takes time. Start out by walking a few minutes each day. Increase the amount of time you walk by 5 minutes each day. After a while you may feel like jogging a little or varying the routine by riding your bike. You build endurance by being a little more physically active each day, by exercising a little longer or a little harder each time. Endurance activities help keep your heart and lungs healthy and also relieve stress and relax the body.

Strength

Many athletes, both boys and girls, include activities that help build and tone muscles in their exercise programs. Weight training is one way to make your muscles work harder to build strength. You can start by lifting light weights—small dumbbells or even books or cans of food. If you want to increase the weight or use weight machines, be sure to get advice from a physical education teacher or coach first.

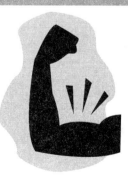

© ETR

Name _____

Physical Activity for Me

Directions: List at least two activities you enjoy or would like to try that build each of the different kinds of fitness and answer the questions. Then think about the good things you get from being active and list your top 5.

Flexibility 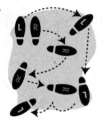	**Endurance** 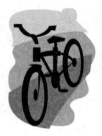	**Strength** 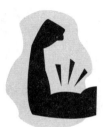

How much physical activity do fifth graders need each day?

_____

What are some things you could do to warm up before and cool down after being physically active?

_____

_____

_____

My Top 5 Benefits of Physical Activity

1. _____

2. _____

3. _____

4. _____

5. _____

_____

Let's Get Moving!

Leticia

Leticia is an active kid. Each morning she rides her bike 20 minutes to get to school and 20 minutes to get home in the afternoon. During recess she likes to play tetherball with a group of friends, and she plays on the city soccer league 3 days a week and 1 day on the weekend.

She stays active at home too. Leticia walks her little brother to the park to play. She works hard washing cars at her church's carwash fundraiser and volunteers to lead outdoor games at the youth club. She's also saving her money to take karate classes. Where does Leticia get all her energy? From exercising and having a healthy body!

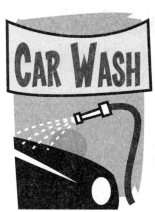

Anthony

Anthony hates exercise...or does he? Today he forged a note from his parents to excuse himself from participating in the school Fitness Fair. Anthony prefers to do other things. He loves to read. He's a whiz on the computer and a video game champ. He spends his lunchtime helping in the school computer lab, and the other students admire his skills.

Anthony felt bad about the note and went for a long walk with his dad to talk about it. At the end of the walk he felt a lot better. He liked how it felt to be moving his body. The physical activity even made his mind feel sharper when he sat down to do his homework. Anthony decided to try walking the next day too.

Questions

1. **What are some ways to add physical activity to your day? Give some examples.**

2. **The story says that Leticia gets energy from exercising and having a healthy body. What do you think this means? What are other positive outcomes of being active?**

3. **How do you think Anthony's story will end? How could he continue to add physical activity and exercise to his day while still doing the other things he likes to do? How hard is it to break old habits or start new ones?**

Name _____

Adding Up My Physical Activity

Part 1

Directions: Write down the amount of physical activity you get in an average day.

Physical Activity	Number of Minutes	Type of Activity
Before School		☐ Aerobic ☐ Flexibility ☐ Strength
During School		☐ Aerobic ☐ Flexibility ☐ Strength
After School		☐ Aerobic ☐ Flexibility ☐ Strength
	Total Number of Minutes: _____	

Part 2

1. What could you do to add more physical activity and exercise in your day?

   _____

   _____

   _____

2. Why is it important to choose different ways to be active?

   _____

   _____

   _____

3. List 3 positive outcomes of physical activity:

   _____

   _____

   _____

Healthy Eating and Physical Activity: Getting Started

1. What is your healthy eating or physical activity goal? _____

_____

_____

2. What will be the benefits of reaching your goal? _____

_____

_____

3. Why is this goal important to you? _____

_____

_____

4. What must you do to reach this goal? _____

_____

_____

5. How will you start? _____

_____

_____

6. Who can help you? _____

_____

_____

7. What could get in the way of reaching your goal?

Barrier	**How I Could Overcome It**
_____	_____
_____	_____
_____	_____
_____	_____

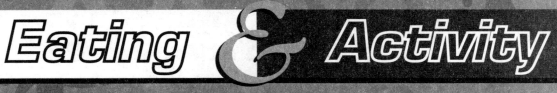

Eating & Activity

Tracking Your Progress

If you were going on a trip, you'd probably do some things before you left. You'd decide where and when you wanted to go, choose which way to go, and plan ahead for what might go wrong. Smart travelers think ahead of time about possible problems and ways to solve them. They also keep in mind the fun they will have along the way.

Like planning a trip, you can plan a physical activity or healthy eating program. You need to know where you want to go. You need to know the benefits of getting there. You need to think ahead of time about what might go wrong and where you could get help. You need to keep track of your progress.

The purpose of planning ahead is to make sure you get where you want to go. Keeping track of your progress can help keep you motivated. Here are some examples.

© ETR

Jamie's Goal *Jamie set a goal to build up to 60 minutes of activity a day.*

Monday

What steps did you take today to meet your goal?
I walked to school this morning and walked quickly on the way back home in the afternoon.

What problem or barrier got in the way today?
I had to stay inside during lunch to work on a project for class, so I wasn't able to play soccer.

What did you do to overcome it?
I decided to exercise at lunch tomorrow.

Who helped you with your goal today?
My friend walked home with me.

Tuesday

What steps did you take today to meet your goal?
I jumped rope—Double Dutch—for all of recess.

What problem or barrier got in the way today?
My friends didn't want to jump rope.

What did you do to overcome it?
I talked them into playing. I told them it would be fun.

Who helped you with your goal today?
My friends agreed to play.

What I Learned This Week

Things I did well:
I was more aware of moving my body and being active, even if I didn't get all the exercise I'd planned.

Benefits I enjoyed this week:
I got to visit with a friend on the walk home on Monday. I had more energy.

Problems I had and how I can solve them:
I've got to plan around special class projects that mean giving up lunchtime exercise. I could do some of the work at home the night before.

What I am going to do toward my goal this weekend:
I'm going on a bike ride with my friends on Saturday.

Niko's Goal *Niko set a goal to build up to eating 2 cups of fruit and 3 cups of vegetables a day.*

Monday

What steps did you take today to meet your goal?
I brought an apple and carrot sticks in my lunch.

Was there a problem or barrier?
I have to clean and prepare the fruits and vegetables for each day.

What did you do to overcome it?
I chose vegetables that were easy to fix (red or green peppers, broccoli, carrots, peas in the pod, cauliflower and celery).

Did anyone help you with your goal today?
My father helped me shop for the vegetables for the entire week.

Tuesday

What steps did you take today to meet your goal?
I put strawberries on my cereal this morning, and had carrot sticks for a snack after school.

Was there a problem or barrier?
I really wanted to eat some cookies after school.

What did you do to overcome it?
I remembered my goal and ate some carrot sticks and one cookie.

Did anyone help you with your goal today?
My dad bought the strawberries.

What I Learned This Week

Things I did well:
I did pretty well. On six of the seven days I ate at least 2 cups of vegetables and 1 ½ cups of fruit.

Benefits I enjoyed this week:
I felt proud that I reached my goal.

Problems I had and how I can solve them:
I get tired of the same fruits. I need to try some other kinds—maybe a mango, plum or apricot.

What I am going to do toward my goal this weekend:
Saturday morning I'm going to prepare some vegetables to snack on during the weekend.

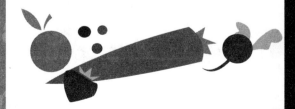

Tracking My Progress

Directions: Complete the questions for each day of the week. On Friday, answer the questions about what you learned this week.

Monday

What steps did you take today to meet your goal?

What problem or barrier got in the way today?

What did you do to overcome it?

Who helped you with your goal today?

Tuesday

What steps did you take today to meet your goal?

What problem or barrier got in the way today?

What did you do to overcome it?

Who helped you with your goal today?

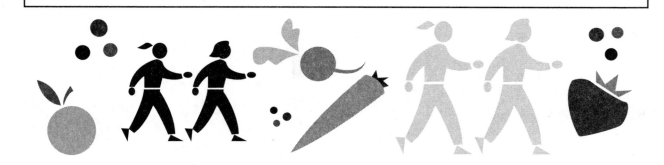

© ETR

Tracking My Progress

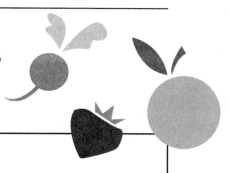

Wednesday

What steps did you take today to meet your goal?

What problem or barrier got in the way today?

What did you do to overcome it?

Who helped you with your goal today?

Thursday

What steps did you take today to meet your goal?

What problem or barrier got in the way today?

What did you do to overcome it?

Who helped you with your goal today?

Friday

What steps did you take today to meet your goal?

What problem or barrier got in the way today?

What did you do to overcome it?

Who helped you with your goal today?

© ETR

Tracking My Progress

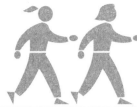

What I Learned This Week

Things I did well: _____

_____

_____

_____

_____

Benefits I enjoyed this week: _____

_____

_____

_____

_____

Problems I had and how I solved them: _____

_____

_____

_____

_____

What I am going to do toward my goal this weekend: _____

_____

_____

_____

_____

© ETR

5 Things I Like to Do

Part 1

Directions: Make a list of 5 things you enjoy doing. You will come back to this list later.

1. _____
2. _____
3. _____
4. _____
5. _____

Part 2

Directions: Explain how using alcohol would affect each of the things you like to do.

1. _____
2. _____
3. _____
4. _____
5. _____

Part 3

Directions: Write how experimenting with alcohol could affect your life. Then share your ideas with a partner.

© ETR

Alcohol and the Body—Right Side

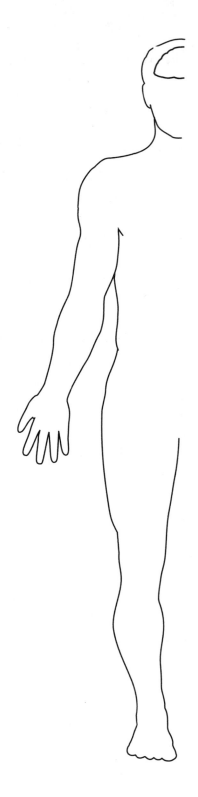

© ETR

Alcohol and the Body—Left Side

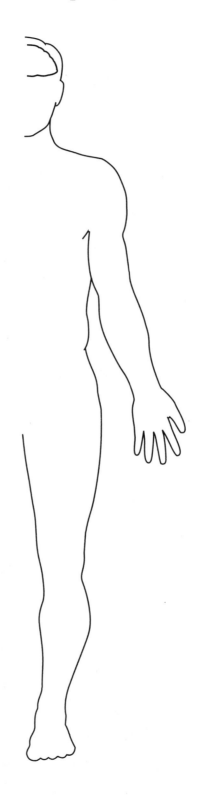

Alcohol & Feelings

Making the Connection

Grounded

My name is Kiet. I'm in eighth grade. I want to tell you about what happened to me so it won't happen to you.

I got grounded because I went out after school with friends without telling my mom where I'd be. I stayed out longer than I should have, but I didn't think it was a reason to be grounded. Mom didn't see it that way. She said nothing but chores and homework for the whole weekend—no TV, no friends, no telephone, no fun! Friday afternoon I went straight home from school but Mom wasn't there. There was a note reminding me I was grounded, and a list of chores to do.

I went into the kitchen to get a snack before starting on the chores. I had to move a six-pack of beer to get to the sandwich stuff in the refrigerator. I decided to try one of the beers. I thought, "Why not? I'm having a bad day. People on TV always have a drink when they're having a bad day. Maybe it will make those chores easier."

The beer didn't taste that good, but it was cold and fizzy, and I started feeling kind of relaxed. I finished the sandwich and decided to drink another beer. Then I went outside to start on the chores, but I started to feel a little dizzy, so I sat down in a lawn chair for a minute. Before I knew it I was waking up to see Mom standing over me, holding an empty beer can. I was sure she was going to be really mad, but it was worse—she just looked sad and disappointed. She told me to go to my room, that we'd talk later. I had a terrible headache that night and my stomach didn't feel good either.

Mom and I talked it out the next day. I told her I was sorry. I couldn't really explain why I drank the beer—I was just mad, I guess. I can tell Mom is still worried about me. Oh, and I'm grounded for two weeks now, so drinking just made it worse!

1. **What did Kiet's feelings have to do with drinking the beer?**
2. **How did Kiet think the beer would help change his feelings?**
3. **How did Kiet feel after drinking?**
4. **How might Kiet have handled the feelings more positively?**

© ETR

Feelings & the Alcohol Connection

Jenny and Me

Jenny and I are in seventh grade. We're best friends. I want to tell you about what happened to us so it won't happen to you.

Jenny came over to spend the night last Saturday. My parents went to bed early, but we were allowed to stay up to watch movies. In this movie there was a scene of college kids partying and drinking beer and stuff. So Jenny and I got out wine glasses, poured our sodas into them, and pretended we were drinking, too. We toasted each other and started acting as if we were drunk.

Then we decided to try a little real alcohol. We went to the liquor cabinet and took a sip from one of the bottles. It tasted bad, so we mixed some with our sodas. That helped the alcohol taste better. We were having fun toasting each other and acting goofy, when all of a sudden we felt sick.

We both ran to the bathroom and threw up. That woke up my parents. They quickly figured out that we'd been drinking. My mom called Jenny's mom to come get her. Mom made me clean up the bathroom even though I still felt sick. She said she certainly wasn't going to clean up the mess.

Now Jenny and I aren't allowed to see each other except at school. Our parents don't trust our judgment when we're together. Mom won't let me stay home alone anymore either. I have to go on all her boring errands with her. She even has the next-door neighbor watch me when she goes out. Seventh grade, and I have to have a babysitter! I'd die if anyone found out. Mom says it will be a while before I earn her trust again.

1. What feelings did the girls have that made them decide to try alcohol?

_____

_____

2. What were the consequences of the girls drinking alcohol?

_____

_____

3. How could they have dealt with the feelings in a positive way?

_____

_____

_____

_____

Feelings & the Alcohol Connection

(continued)

A.J.

My name is A.J. I'm in ninth grade. I want to tell you about what happened to me. Some of you might be in a similar situation. I hope you make a different choice than I did.

Last week my dad busted me and my friends when we got into his liquor cabinet and drank some of the liquor. We got sick, and one of my friends threw up all over my dad's pool table. Dad was furious with me. After my friends' parents came to get them, he came to my room and wanted to know why I'd pulled a stunt like that.

I was silent for a long time. Then I said, "Remember the fishing trip we were supposed to go on last weekend? You had a business meeting to get ready for and you had to cancel—again. Remember my swim meet two weeks ago? It was my last meet of the year and you promised to be there. You weren't. I guess I was mad at you."

Dad listened quietly. Then he said, "A.J., I'm still angry with you for getting into the liquor. But obviously we need to spend some more time talking. I know it's been hard since your mom left, and I don't have as much time to spend with you. But alcohol isn't the way to deal with your problems."

1. What feelings did A.J. have that led to drinking alcohol?

   _____

   _____

2. What were the consequences of A.J. and friends drinking alcohol?

   _____

   _____

3. How could A.J. have dealt with the feelings in a positive way?

   _____

   _____

   _____

   _____

Alcohol & Peers

Rochelle

Every summer my family goes on a camping trip to the same lake. There are usually some other kids staying at the lake. Most of them are a couple of years older than I am. They like to hang out in the evenings listening to CDs and drinking.

One night I wanted some company, so I decided I'd join the crowd. The kids were friendly but I wasn't there five minutes before I was offered a beer. I said, "No, thanks," and they pretty much left it at that—except for this one kid. He wanted to know why I wouldn't drink with them. I was embarrassed to say I'd promised my parents not to drink until I was 21, so I just said I didn't like the taste of beer.

He started hassling me, telling me nobody liked beer the first time they tried it, that I should give it another chance. "Try this," he said. "I guarantee you'll like it. It's the good stuff." I suddenly felt as if I was on stage, that everyone was watching to see what I'd do. So I said OK and took one of the green bottles. I thought I'd just hold it and they'd leave me alone, but then he said, "OK, let's see you take a swig of it before it gets warm."

Everybody was watching to see what I'd do. I took a gulp. "So how was that?" he asked. "Good," I lied. Actually, I'd hardly tasted the beer at all. All I could think of was that I broke a promise I'd made to my parents just to impress a kid I'd probably never see again.

Back at our campsite, my mom asked if I'd had a good time and I said I had. But then she moved closer and gave me a funny look. "You've been drinking," she said. "I thought you promised not to."

1. **Why did Rochelle drink the beer?**
2. **What are some examples of peer pressure in the story?**
3. **How could Rochelle have avoided or resisted the pressure?**
4. **How do you think this story ended?**

Peers & the Alcohol Connection

Adrian

Roman is my best friend. He's probably the most popular kid at our middle school. Roman is a good student, a starter on our school's basketball team, and a really great artist. Everybody likes Roman—kids, teachers, parents, the janitors—everybody. And what makes Roman different from many other popular kids is that he treats everyone like a friend. I really admire him.

We were at a party last weekend and somebody had beer they'd swiped from home. One kid asked Roman if he wanted a beer and Roman said, "Sure." I was really surprised, because it's basketball season and I know how serious Roman is about playing ball—he's already been scouted by high school coaches in our town and he's hoping to make varsity as a freshman. I asked Roman why he'd damage his reputation by messing around with alcohol. The way kids gossip at our school, if you have one beer, next you hear you had ten.

Roman just smiled and said, "What's the big deal? Everybody else is doing it. It's just one or two beers." So I took a beer too.

1. Why did Adrian and Roman drink?

   _____

   _____

2. What are some examples of peer pressure in the story?

   _____

   _____

3. How could Adrian and Roman have avoided or resisted the pressure?

   _____

   _____

4. Write a new ending for the story in which peers are a positive influence and help Adrian and/or Roman choose not to drink alcohol.

   _____

   _____

   _____

   _____

© ETR

Alcohol & the Media

BUY!

Making the Connection

Wisecracking lizards, football-loving horses, beautiful people in swimsuits playing volleyball on the beach, fans in the stands watching the game. What do all these images have in common? They've all been used to advertise beer. Think about the television ads you can remember. Chances are, some of them are beer commercials. Many beer ads are clever, funny and include memorable characters.

In another popular technique to sell their product, advertisers show attractive young people laughing and having a good time playing sports, running on the beach or sailing—and drinking beer. But does this make sense? If beer drinkers are so active, where did the expression "beer belly" come from?

New beer commercials and advertising campaigns are often introduced during major sporting broadcasts. In fact, beer commercials often stand out as the most entertaining. It costs over $5 million to show just one 30-second ad during the Super Bowl—that's a great deal of money to link drinking beer with having fun.

Movies, TV shows and music videos also send messages about alcohol use. Drinking is sometimes shown as a way to loosen up and have fun. The negative effects are rarely shown. But using alcohol greatly increases the chances of getting into a fight, being in a car crash, or being arrested. Over 30% of motor vehicle-related deaths involve alcohol. And remember the fun-loving beer drinkers at the beach? Drinking alcohol plays a role in up to 70% of deaths associated with water recreation.

1. Why might certain ads for alcohol appeal to kids?

2. What don't the ads tell you about alcohol?

7 Ways to Resist Pressure

1. **Say NO and say nothing else.** When someone pressures you, simply say no.

2. **Use body language that says no too.** Be sure your gestures and tone of voice reinforce the NO.

3. **Keep saying NO.** If the pressure continues, repeat the word No.

4. **Give a reason.** Explain why you choose to refuse. "I have an allergy" or "My mom would kill me."

5. **Leave the situation.** As soon as you feel pressured, leave. Don't wait a minute longer.

6. **Suggest something else to do.** "How about shooting a few baskets?" or "I'm on my way to the library. Want to come?"

7. **Ignore the problem.** Change the subject or pretend you didn't hear.

Peer Resistance in Action

Here are some examples of how kids like you resisted peer pressure. Which way was used in each situation?

Example 1

My best friend stole some of his father's beer. He asked me if I wanted to try one. I told him no. When he asked why not, I said, "Look, if it tastes as bad as it smells, forget it."

Example 2

I don't know how we ended up at this party where everyone was way older than us and drinking, but there we were! This guy came over to talk to us. He started offering me and my friend a drink. We kept saying no and he kept pressuring us.

Finally, I told the guy that the reason that I didn't drink was that my mom was coming to pick me up and she'd be really mad if she smelled alcohol on my breath. I know he thought we were wimps but at least he left us alone.

Example 3

This girl I know once tried to talk me into smoking crack with her. She said it was the best high there is. I told her that crack was addictive and that it can mess your heart up. And then I got out of there, *fast*.

Example 4

This older kid asked my friend and me if we wanted to drink some beer after school. Before my friend could answer, I said, "No. Let's go shoot some hoops over at my house instead." My friend said OK, and that's what we did.

Example 5

I went over to my friend's house so we could work on our project for the health fair together. We were down in the basement, putting our model together, when my friend got a bottle of alcohol from the cupboard and offered me some.

I asked, "What are you doing?" My friend told me that drinking would relax us and make us more creative. I said, "No way. Not in a million years." I said to put the bottle back or to get another partner.

© ETR

Group Plan for Resisting Alcohol Pressures

Directions: Read your group's situation. Answer these questions to prepare for the roleplay.

What do we need to say and when? _____

_____

_____

To whom do we need to say it? _____

_____

What words will we use? _____

_____

What body language will we use? _____

_____

What reason could we give? _____

_____

_____

_____

What alternative could we suggest? _____

_____

_____

_____

Name _____

Alcohol Free: One Choice at a Time

Directions: Read the story. Then go through the steps to make a healthy choice.

You and a friend are walking home after school and find an unopened bottle of alcohol next to a garbage can. Your friend thinks it would be fun to try some and find out what it feels like to get drunk.

What decision do you need to make?

What are your choices?

1.

What could happen with this choice?	
+ positive consequences	**–** negative consequences

2.

What could happen with this choice?	
+ positive consequences	**–** negative consequences

(continued)

© ETR

Alcohol Free: One Choice at a Time

(continued)

3.

What could happen with this choice?	
+ positive consequences	**−** negative consequences

Do you need help with this choice?

☐ YES   ☐ NO

Who can help you?

What's the healthy choice for you? Why?

© ETR

Name _____

A Closer Look at Me and Alcohol Connections

Directions: Read the questions and select a "yes" or "no" response for each. Use the last column to describe evidence of your own personal behavior that supports your answer. then circle the 3 things that will most help you stay alcohol free.

Statements		My Evidence

Choices and Consequences

Do I believe that being alcohol free is a
smart and safe choice for me? ☐ yes ☐ no _____

Do I understand how using alcohol
could increase the risk of being injured? ☐ yes ☐ no _____

Do I believe that using alcohol could get me in
trouble with the law? ☐ yes ☐ no _____

Do I believe that using alcohol could negatively
affect my reputation? ☐ yes ☐ no _____

Feelings

Do I have healthy ways to deal with
strong emotions (sadness, disappointment, anger)? ☐ yes ☐ no _____

Do I have healthy things to do when I'm bored? ☐ yes ☐ no _____

Do I feel good enough about myself to not drink alcohol? ☐ yes ☐ no _____

Do I believe that drinking alcohol makes problems worse? ☐ yes ☐ no _____

Peers

Do I have friends who expect me to be alcohol free? ☐ yes ☐ no _____

Do I have healthy ways of dealing with
peer pressure to drink alcohol? ☐ yes ☐ no _____

Can I influence others (use peer power) to be alcohol free? ☐ yes ☐ no _____

Do I believe that being alcohol free is
part of a good reputation? ☐ yes ☐ no _____

Media

Do I understand that the goal of alcohol ads is to
persuade people to drink? ☐ yes ☐ no _____

Do I understand that the media tries to make drinking
alcohol look exciting, glamorous and fun? ☐ yes ☐ no _____

Do I believe that alcohol companies pay filmmakers to
use their products in movies? ☐ yes ☐ no _____

Do I ask myself if media messages about alcohol
are true or complete? ☐ yes ☐ no _____

I, _____ , choose to be alcohol free because: _____
    (name)

Alcohol-Free Road Map

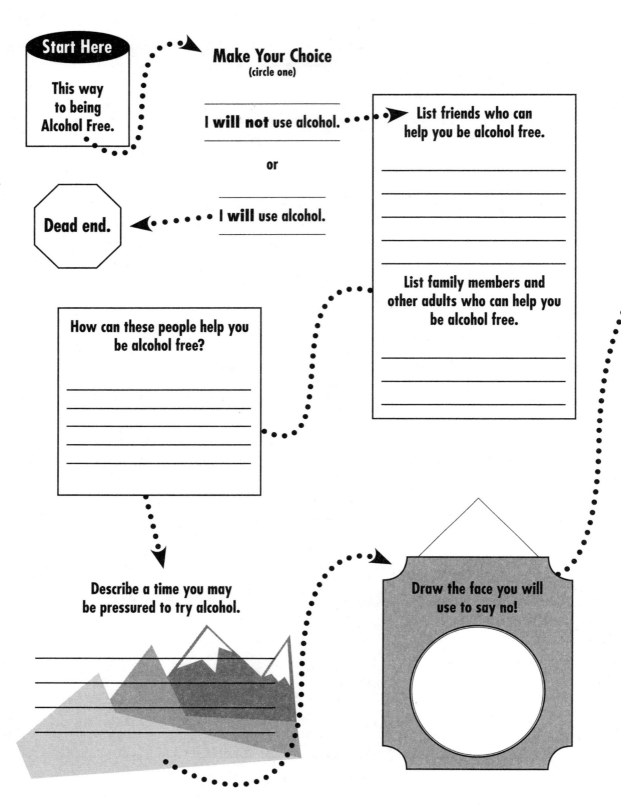

Start Here

This way to being Alcohol Free.

Make Your Choice
(circle one)

_____
I **will not** use alcohol.

or

_____
I **will** use alcohol.

Dead end.

List friends who can help you be alcohol free.

_____
_____
_____
_____
_____

List family members and other adults who can help you be alcohol free.

_____
_____
_____

How can these people help you be alcohol free?

_____
_____
_____
_____
_____

Describe a time you may be pressured to try alcohol.

_____
_____
_____
_____

Draw the face you will use to say no!

© ETR

(continued)

Alcohol-Free Road Map
(continued)

List the words you will use to say no to pressure.

_____
_____
_____
_____
_____
_____
_____

How can the media influence choices about alcohol?

_____
_____
_____

Consequences

List other things in your life that could be affected by alcohol use.

_____
_____
_____
_____
_____

Name 3 things that can happen to your body if you use alcohol.

_____
_____
_____

Consequences

Outcomes.
Describe what will happen if you choose to be alcohol free.

_____
_____
_____
_____

YOU ARE HERE!

Draw a picture of alcohol-free you.

SPECIAL AND VERY SMART PERSON.

© ETR

WHEN OTHERS DRINK

Cody

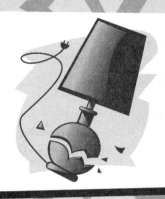

At Cody's house, Friday nights are the worst. Every Friday night Cody's dad drinks an entire case of beer. He starts drinking right after dinner and doesn't stop until sometime around midnight. The family has learned to leave Cody's father alone when he's drinking. Sometimes he gets angry or violent and will pick a fight over nothing. He throws things and smashes furniture. Other times he just gets sad and depressed. He drinks in the dark with the TV on until he passes out.

Christina

Christina's mother is like two different people. One of them is a nice, normal mom, and the other is mean, nasty and sarcastic. When Christina's mom drinks, her whole personality changes. Christina's mom has said some terrible things when she's had too much to drink. She's called Christina "stupid," "ugly," "worthless" and worse. Christina tries her best to believe her mom doesn't really mean the things she says when she's been drinking—that it's the alcohol talking—but it still hurts.

Roberto

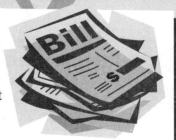

Roberto will never forget the time his father hit his mother. His father had been drinking and arguing with his mom about the bills. The argument got louder and louder, until Roberto's father jumped up and hit Roberto's mother hard, knocking her down on the kitchen floor. Roberto jumped between them and tried to protect his mom. He was scared. Roberto's father is a big man—over 6 feet tall—and Roberto is only 13.

© ETR

JAY

Jay should be used to waiting by now, but it still makes him upset and angry. His mother promised to pick up Jay and his friends at the mall at 5:30. Now it's 6:15. It's getting cold and dark and Jay's mom is still nowhere to be seen. Jay's trying to keep his cool in front of his friends, but as each minute ticks by he's becoming more and more upset. "She probably stopped at a bar after work for a drink," Jay thinks. "Why can't I ever count on her to be on time?"

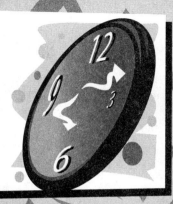

ERICA

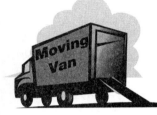

Erica's father has lost another job. It's the same old story—he was fired for showing up late and for missing too many days of work. Erica's father has a hard time getting up in the morning because he's a heavy drinker. Erica and her mother have asked him to cut down on his drinking and to get some help for his problem. But nothing ever seems to change. Now Erica and her family will probably have to move to a less expensive apartment.

ANDREW

Andrew is only 13 but sometimes he thinks he's the only adult living in his house. In the morning, he gets his brother and sister up and ready for school. He helps them make their lunches, feeds the dog and takes out the trash. After school, he does his homework and then starts dinner. Andrew does laundry, cleans the house and does yardwork. When there is no food in the house, he has to nag his parents to go to the supermarket.

When his P.E. teacher asked him to try out for the middle school basketball team, Andrew was thrilled—he wanted more than anything to play for the team. But he had to say no when he realized that the team would practice every day after school for two hours. Who would look after his brother and sister? Who would make sure there was food and clean clothes? Andrew's teacher couldn't understand why Andrew said no. Andrew thought, "If you knew my parents were alcoholics, maybe you'd understand."

The kids in these stories all share a similar problem: They live with a family member who is using and abusing alcohol. Kids in these situations are in a terrible bind. Sometimes they blame themselves for their parents' problems. Sometimes they try to cover up the problem by pretending it doesn't exist or by taking on way more responsibility than they should have to. And very often they live in a state of constant fear—fear of violence, verbal abuse, abandonment, embarrassment and poverty. It's hard to say what's worse: being an alcoholic or living with one.

Real Stories:
Getting Help When Others Drink

In Charge

I can't remember a time when I haven't been in charge. My mom is an alcoholic. She manages to go to work every day, but when she gets home she starts drinking. I do the shopping and the laundry, and I cook dinner and help my little brother with his homework. Every morning I make sure we get up and go to school. I bring mom her coffee and try to make sure she goes to work. Dad isn't around much. He and mom got a divorce a few years ago and he lives in another state. Until recently, life was OK. I was used to being the responsible one.

But then my little brother started to get into trouble at school. He fought with other kids and wouldn't come home after school. His grades were dropping. It got harder for me to handle him, too. The school would call my mom, but she never kept her appointments with the teacher. One evening my brother's teacher called. Mom was already out of it, so I said she was sick. The teacher asked if I could stop by school the next day to see her. I said sure. I had to do something about my brother.

The next day when I got there, I was surprised to find my brother there too. He confessed that he had told his teacher all about our mom and her drinking. At first I was very angry because we had always kept this a secret. It was embarrassing to have a mom who didn't do the mom stuff because she was drunk all the time. But after a while it was a relief to know that someone else knew. Being in charge was getting to be too hard.

My brother and I both cried and talked and his teacher listened. She said she couldn't change our situation, but she could listen and try to get someone to help us. Right now that feels good, because I've never really had anyone to talk to. I'm glad the secret is out.

© ETR

My Brother

I love my brother. I hate my brother. My brother is messing up our whole family. Jeff used to be a cool big brother. We'd fight sometimes and he'd tease me, but I could always count on him to be there for me. Not anymore. He's more interested in going out with friends and drinking. My parents don't even seem to know I'm around now. If Dad isn't yelling, he doesn't talk at all, and Mom cries all the time. There's always some new crisis with my brother.

About a month ago my brother really blew it. He and some friends were drinking and they stole a car and crashed it. My brother was driving. Luckily no one was hurt badly, but he got arrested. Now my parents have to come up with the money for a lawyer. My brother takes all their attention. I even thought I was going to have to quit the basketball team because I could never count on anyone to take me to practice.

I talked to my coach and told him I didn't think I could stay on the team. He asked me what was going on, and said he'd noticed I seemed moody and depressed. I guess he caught me off guard—I actually told him about my brother and his drinking and how angry I was with my parents for ignoring me.

Coach was really cool. He told me his dad had been an alcoholic—that's what they call someone who's addicted to alcohol—and that it really messed up his family too. Coach told me about a group that helped him cope. It's called Alateen, where kids with family members who are alcoholic get together and talk. Coach is going to help me find an Alateen group here. He also said he was available to talk and that he'd make sure I get to practice. He even offered to talk to my parents. I can't do anything about my brother's problems and his drinking, but it's great to know I have someone to talk to.

The Car Wreck That Changed My Life

Last year I was in a car wreck that changed my life—for the better! I wouldn't have thought so at the time, but that crash started some big changes in my family. We had gone to my dad's company picnic. It was great at first—lots of food and games and seeing people. But then Dad started to drink, and once he starts he can't seem to stop. By the time the picnic was over, Dad was drunk. Mom tried to take the car keys away from him, but he insisted he was OK.

We were all a little nervous about getting into the car with Dad, but he'd never crashed before so we all hoped it would be OK. Dad was fine at first. He drove slowly, and since it had been a long day I dozed off in the back seat. I woke up to the sound of screeching brakes. My dad had run a stop sign and we just missed hitting another car. Our car ran up the curb and hit a mailbox. Luckily none of us were badly hurt, but we had to go to the hospital anyway.

At the hospital, the police came and arrested my dad for drunk driving. They said we were very lucky no one was killed. A doctor had a long talk with my mom and gave her some pamphlets about living with an alcoholic. When we got home she talked about what the doctor had said to her. She and I started going to meetings where people can talk about living with an alcoholic.

Dad got out of jail. He can't drive anymore because the judge took his license away. He still drinks. Mom and I can't do anything about that, but it helps that we can talk about it together and in our groups. I even found some other kids at school who have parents who are alcoholics too. It's still hard to have a dad who's an alcoholic, but now I know I'm the only person I can control.

Kids Like You

Fernando Fernando has always been close to his family. But now that he's in fifth grade, he finds it hard at times to choose between family and friends. Fernando loves his family—he just wants to hang out with other kids his own age.

What do you think Fernando might be feeling?

_____

Samantha Samantha wonders if the new boy in her class will talk to her today. He seems very quiet and shy—he's been there for two weeks and has hardly said a word to anyone. But Samantha likes him and thinks he likes her.

What do you think Samantha and the new boy might be feeling?

_____

LeRoy LeRoy's dad tells him that growing up happens fast enough without rushing it. His dad says that there will be plenty of time for LeRoy to do the things he wants. But LeRoy's friends give him a hard time when he doesn't get to do the things they do or go to some of the places they go.

What do you think LeRoy might be feeling?

_____

Bill His older brother is 5'10" and Bill hopes he will get to be at least that tall. Bill hates being the shortest boy on the basketball team. He'd really like to play another position besides guard. All the girls at school call him "cute"—as if he's a puppy or something.

What do you think Bill might be feeling?

_____

Jayla Jayla's parents can be a little strict at times. Jayla gets jealous of friends who get to make more choices than she does. Her friends seem to have more say about the clothes they wear and the things they do. Jayla would like to try wearing a little makeup, but she's not sure her parents would go for that.

What do you think Jayla might be feeling?

_____

© ETR

Puberty and My Feelings

Directions: Complete the checklist. Which of these feelings have you had?

___ shy	___ curious	___ frustrated
___ angry	___ jealous	___ lonely
___ embarrassed	___ accepted	___ had a crush on someone
___ happy	___ rejected	___ am I normal?
___ independent	___ confused	___ other _____
___ scared	___ stressed	___ other _____

Choose one of the feelings from the list and write about a time you felt this way.

_____

_____

_____

_____

_____

_____

_____

_____

_____

_____

_____

© ETR

Name _____

Old Me, New Me

Directions: Read and complete the chart.

Ways I Have Changed

	What's different about me now	Why I like or don't like the change
Socially (my friends)		
Mentally (my thoughts)		
Physically (my body)		
Emotionally (my feelings)		

© ETR